COMPLETE GUIDE TO DUPUYTREN'S CONTRACTURE SURGERY

Comprehensive Manual To Advanced Techniques, Recovery, and Best Practices for Optimal Oral Health

DR. BRUNO HORAN

Disclaimer:

The information provided in this book, is intended for general informational purposes only and should not be considered as professional advice.

The author has made every effort to ensure the accuracy of the information presented. However, readers are advised to consult with a qualified healthcare professional before attempting any herbal remedies or making significant changes to their wellness routine. Individual health conditions vary, and what may be suitable for one person may not be appropriate for another.

It is important to note that the author is not in any endorsement deal, partnership, or affiliation with any organization, brand, or company mentioned in this book. Any references to specific products or services are based on the author's personal experience or general knowledge and do not imply an

endorsement or promotion of those products or
services

Contents

For anyone dealing with this condition, "Dupuytren's Contracture Surgery" is a vital resource that provides a thorough overview of, guidance during, and recuperation following surgical therapy. The book walks patients through the initial consultations and necessary evaluations in its first section, which focuses on the preparatory phase. It emphasizes how crucial it is to provide patients with preoperative information and expectations management, as informed patients are better able to manage their surgery experience and recuperation. Careful planning for the recovery period following surgery guarantees that patients know what to anticipate and how best to handle their convalescence.

Investigating different surgical techniques is especially beneficial. The book goes into detail on the subtleties of needle aponeurotomy (NA), the application of collagenase injections (Xiaflex), and the distinctions between fasciotomy and fasciectomy. Additionally, it presents cutting-edge methods and research, giving patients and medical professionals a better understanding of recent developments. A patient-centric approach is reflected in the emphasis on selecting the best method based on each patient's unique circumstances, guaranteeing individualized and efficient treatment regimens.

A thorough, step-by-step explanation of the surgical procedure demystifies the procedure by elucidating the various anesthetic alternatives, incision methods, and wound closure procedures.

 Along with discussing the usual recovery period and crucial post-operative care, the book also covers potential difficulties and how to treat them. Patients gain knowledge from this segment, which lowers their worry and increases their sense of readiness.

It is imperative to comprehend the advantages and disadvantages, and the book is forthright in addressing typical surgical risks, long-term consequences, and the effectiveness of alternate therapies. Testimonials from patients and patient satisfaction rates provide practical insights, highlighting the significance of follow-up treatment in getting the best outcomes.

Recovery and rehabilitation receive a great deal of attention, along with comprehensive guidance on pain management techniques, physical therapy, and immediate postoperative care.

A comprehensive approach to rehabilitation is ensured through the instructions for going back to regular activities and jobs, as well as monitoring progress and any difficulties.

Following surgery, changing one's lifestyle is essential to preserving hand health and avoiding recurrence. The book offers helpful advice on daily hand workouts, ergonomic hand use, and adapted tools in addition to nutritional and lifestyle suggestions to promote general wellbeing.

Surgery's psychological and emotional effects are taken into consideration. The book discusses how to manage stress and anxiety, how it affects confidence and self-image, and how crucial support networks are. It provides a comprehensive approach to patient care by taking mental health issues into account while the patient is recovering.

The story is enhanced by real-world case studies and patient experiences, which provide a range of viewpoints and helpful guidance from both patients and medical professionals. The lessons and insights these stories offer make the book an accessible and educational read.

Last but not least, the FAQs section answers frequently asked questions concerning Dupuytren's contracture causes, if surgery is necessary, alternative treatments, recovery times, and expected hand function after surgery. It does this straightforwardly and succinctly. This section ensures that patients have easy access to vital information by acting as a quick reference.

All things considered, "Dupuytren's Contracture Surgery" is a thorough manual that combines medical knowledge with helpful guidance to meet patients' physical, emotional, and psychological requirements.

CHAPTER ONE

GETTING READY FOR SURGERY

First Consultations And Evaluations

The first consultations with your healthcare practitioner are very important when getting ready for surgery to correct Dupuytren's contracture.

Your surgeon will examine you physically and go over your medical history in detail to determine the extent of your condition during these visits.

They will go over the anticipated results, any dangers, and the surgical technique. You can use this time to ask questions and get any doubts you may have regarding the procedure answered.

A successful surgery is mostly dependent on you and your surgeon having a common understanding.

Exams And Assessments Before Surgery

Several examinations and tests are required before having surgery to treat Dupuytren's contracture to make sure you are a good candidate.

It may be necessary to perform blood tests to look for any underlying medical issues that might interfere with healing.

To provide a clear picture of the affected hand and the degree of tissue involvement, imaging tests like X-rays or ultrasounds may be prescribed. These tests assist your surgeon in more accurately planning the procedure and foreseeing any potential difficulties.

Instructions And Preparations For Preoperative Care

In the days preceding your procedure, you will get detailed instructions from your physician regarding preoperative care. These could include restrictions on what can be consumed and eaten, drugs to stay away from, and unique circumstances like quitting smoking to speed up recovery. It can also be suggested that you get your house ready for recovery from surgery by making sure you have comfortable sleeping quarters and easy access to supplies. It is essential that you carefully follow these directions to reduce risks and maximize surgical outcomes.

Taking Care Of Expectations And Worries

It is normal to feel anxious and worried before having surgery. Dealing with these feelings is a crucial step in becoming ready. Your medical staff will assist you in being aware of what to anticipate before, during, and following the surgery.

Setting reasonable expectations can be aided by being aware of the likelihood of pain, the recovery period, and the likely results of the procedure. It might also be helpful to talk about any anxieties you may have with your surgeon or a counselor so that you feel ready both emotionally and cognitively for the procedure.

Organizing Your Recuperation After Surgery

Making good plans for your recovery after surgery is crucial to a seamless and fruitful recovery process. After the procedure, make arrangements for a driver to take you home because anesthesia and painkillers can make it difficult for you to drive.

During the early stages of recuperation, think about scheduling assistance for everyday tasks like cleaning, cooking, and personal hygiene. A thorough rehabilitation plan that includes wound care instructions, physical therapy exercises, and follow-up sessions will be given by your surgeon. Following this strategy religiously will help you go back to your normal functioning level and make the most out of your surgery.

CHAPTER TWO

SURGICAL PROCEDURES TYPES

Fasciectomy Versus Fasciotomy

Fasciotomy and fasciectomy are two popular surgical treatments used to treat Dupuytren's contracture.

Making tiny incisions in the bands of fibrous tissue, called fascia, that cause the fingers to bend inward is known as a fasciotomy. To remove the tension and enable the fingers to straighten, the surgeon cuts through the tightened cords. There is typically less downtime after this operation because it is less intrusive. However, because the diseased tissue is left in situ, there is an increased risk of recurrence.

On the other hand, a fasciectomy entails removing the diseased fascia. This treatment can be performed in several ways: limited fasciectomy, which removes only the afflicted tissue, and radical fasciectomy, which removes all potentially impacted tissue. Although there is a greater chance of problems like nerve injury or infection, this method is more intrusive, requires a longer recovery period, and may be more successful in preventing recurrence.

The decision between the two treatments is based on various considerations, including the degree of contracture, the patient's health, and the likelihood of recurrence. The goal of both surgeries is to enhance finger extension and hand function.

Nauseous Aponeurotomy

A minimally invasive surgery called needle aponeurotomy (NA) is used to treat Dupuytren's contracture. Using a tiny needle, the tissue cord causing the contracture is split and punctured in this method.

The operation can be done in an outpatient setting because it is usually done under local anesthetic. The surgeon repeatedly punctures the cord with the needle to weaken it and make it possible to straighten the finger. Patients with early-stage contractures or those whose health prevents them from undergoing more intrusive surgery can benefit most from NA.

Even while NA has advantages like reduced pain, faster healing, and less scarring, it might not work as well for contractures that affect more than one finger or that are more severe. In addition, compared to more intrusive surgical procedures, there is a greater chance of the contracture recurring.

Injections Of Collagenase (Xiaflex)

Injections of collagenase, sold under the brand name Xiaflex, offer a non-surgical alternative for the treatment of Dupuytren's contracture.

The collagenase clostridium histolyticum enzyme is injected straight into the tissue chord responsible for the contracture as part of this treatment.

The enzyme functions by dissolving the collagen in the cord, weakening it, and facilitating manual manipulation and finger straightening.

A day or two after the injection, the patient usually has a manipulation session where the physician tries to realign the finger.

This procedure can be performed in a doctor's office and is less intrusive than surgery. It also has a lower risk of complications and a quicker recovery period. It might not be appropriate for all patients, particularly those with more severe contractures or those who have had an enzyme allergy. Furthermore, the possibility of a recurrence persists.

New Methods And Studies

New methods and treatments are being investigated in the treatment of Dupuytren's contracture to enhance results and lower recurrence rates.

One new method is lip grafting, which involves injecting the patient's fat cells into the hand. This technique is supposed to offer a cushion that can enhance hand function and lessen the likelihood that the contracture will return.

Stem cell treatment is a subject of additional research. Researchers are looking at the possibility of using stem cells to mend damaged tissue and lessen fibrosis, which could lead to a longer-lasting cure for Dupuytren's contracture.

Additionally under investigation are developments in robotically aided surgery and minimally invasive surgical methods.

These techniques seek to minimize tissue damage, shorten recovery time, and reduce the chance of problems, all while maintaining the precision of traditional surgery.

Selecting The Appropriate Process For Each Case

Making the right treatment choice for Dupuytren's contracture is a unique choice that has to be discussed with a medical expert.

The ideal course of action depends on several variables, including the patient's age, general health, preferences, and the stage and severity of the contracture.

Because of their shorter recovery times and reduced risk profiles, less invasive methods such as collagenase injections or needle aponeurotomy may be used for early-stage contracture. Even though the recovery time is lengthier, a fasciectomy may be required for more severe cases to offer a more permanent cure.

Important factors to take into account are the patient's lifestyle and work requirements. A patient whose profession significantly depends on hand function would be more interested in a technique with the least amount of downtime, whereas another patient might be more interested in reducing the likelihood of recurrence.

In the end, a comprehensive assessment and consultation with a hand specialist can assist in identifying the best course of action and weighing potential risks, effectiveness, and rehabilitation.

CHAPTER THREE

STEP-BY-STEP PROCEDURE FOR SURGERY

Options And Considerations For Anesthesia

One of the first and most crucial choices to be made while having surgery for Dupuytren's Contracture is the kind of anesthetic. There are normally three options: local anesthetic, regional anesthesia, and general anesthesia.

When using local anesthesia, the hand is only numbed in the precise location where the procedure will be performed. It's generally preferable for less severe situations and lets the patient stay awake and conscious during the surgery.

Blocking the nerves in a broader region of the body, like an arm, is known as regional anesthesia. This compromise approach guarantees deeper numbing while maintaining the patient's consciousness and pain tolerance.

General Anesthesia: This option induces a state of controlled unconsciousness in patients, and is used for more involved surgeries or for individuals who would rather not be awake. When more than one finger is involved or the patient is anxious about the treatment, it is usually employed.

The degree of the illness, the patient's health, and personal preferences are some of the variables that influence the anesthetic choice. Based on these factors, the surgeon and anesthesiologist will talk about the best course of action.

Methods Of Making Incisions And Healing Wounds

The surgical team makes the incision after administering the anesthesia. Although the precise method employed may differ, the following are typical strategies:

Open fasciectomy: This conventional method entails cutting a longitudinal incision or zigzag pattern down the palm and afflicted fingers. This makes it possible for the surgeon to reach and cut the thicker bands of tissue that are causing the contracture. Because of the bigger incision, this approach offers clear visibility and access, but it takes longer to recuperate.

Limited Fasciectomy: Using this technique, the surgeon removes only the thickened tissue that is most troublesome by making smaller, more deliberate incisions. This lessens the hand's overall trauma and may hasten the healing process.

Dermofasciectomy: In extreme circumstances, the surgeon may remove the diseased tissue and the skin that covers it, replacing it with a skin transplant. This approach requires more intricate wound care but is intended to stop recurrence.

The incisions are carefully closed by the surgeon after the constricted tissue has been removed. To stop fluid buildup, tiny drainage tubes may occasionally be inserted in addition to sutures or stitches. With great care, the wound is closed to reduce scarring and encourage the best possible healing.

Handling Surgical Complications

Even with careful planning, surgical problems can occur. These could include infection, hemorrhage, or injury to the nerves.

Bleeding: Surgeons are equipped to stop excessive bleeding by applying hemostatic medications to stop the bleeding or by cauterizing blood vessels.

Nerve harm: Accidental harm is possible due to the close closeness of nerves in the hand. Surgeons carefully maneuver around these nerves using devices with exact magnification.

Infection: Surgeons keep their workspace sterile and use prophylactic antibiotics to avoid infection. Any indication of an infection is promptly treated with the necessary care.

To properly manage these potential problems and guarantee the best possible outcomes for the patient, intraoperative monitoring and a highly competent surgical team are essential.

Length And Average Recuperation Period

Depending on the degree of the contracture and the type of surgery performed, the length of a Dupuytren's Contracture procedure can change. The process normally takes 45 minutes to two hours.

Following surgery, patients should anticipate a few hours of recuperation while the anesthetic wears off. Initially, the hand must be elevated and pain and swelling must be managed, usually with medicine.

First Week: To minimize swelling, patients are advised to keep their bandaged hands elevated. To keep your mobility, you could be advised to do some light exercise.

After two to four weeks, the stitches are taken out, and more vigorous physical therapy is frequently started. Patients eventually return to their regular activities, though they are still advised to avoid heavy lifting and hand straining.

Six weeks to three months: During this time, the majority of patients make significant progress. Physical treatment continues to enhance strength and functionality.

It may take several months to fully recover, including for the swelling to go down and for hand function to fully return. The amount of time depends on each patient's rate of recovery and compliance with post-operative care guidelines.

Following Surgery: Monitoring and Care

Good post-operative care is essential for achieving the best possible recovery and avoiding recurrence. Important elements consist of:

Wound Care: It's crucial to maintain a dry and clean surgical site. Usually, dressings are changed regularly, and the healthcare professional is notified right away of any infection-related symptoms like redness or discharge.

Pain Management: Prescription drugs are used to treat pain; in cases of milder suffering, over-the-counter products may be suggested. Pain can also be reduced by keeping the hand raised.

Physical Therapy: Regaining strength and mobility requires performing the exercises that are suggested by a physical therapist.

The intensity of these workouts is designed to increase progressively as the healing process advances.

Monitoring for Complications: The surgeon will schedule routine follow-up sessions to check recovery and quickly address any concerns. We keep a watchful eye out for complications including stiffness, scarring, or contracture recurrence.

To guarantee a seamless and effective recovery, patients are advised to follow all post-operative instructions and stay in constant contact with their healthcare team.

CHAPTER FOUR

RISKS AND ADVANTAGES OF CONTRACTURE SURGERY WITH DUPUYTREN

Typical Hazards Linked To Surgery

The possible dangers associated with surgery for Dupuytren's Contracture must be understood. Several common hazards associated with surgical intervention include bleeding, infection, and anesthesia-related side effects. In particular, there is a chance of hand nerve or blood vessel injury following Dupuytren's Contracture surgery, which could lead to either temporary or permanent numbness or weakness. Another issue is the creation of scar tissue, which can cause the fingers to become stiff or less mobile.

After surgery, the contracture may reoccur in certain individuals, requiring additional care. Furthermore, problems like prolonged pain or delayed wound healing are conceivable, especially if the patient has underlying medical conditions like diabetes or poor circulation. Patients can more effectively assess the advantages of surgery against the possibility of problems by being aware of these risks.

Long-Term Gains And Results

Dupuytren's Contracture surgery has major long-term benefits for many patients, despite the dangers. By releasing the tightened tissues, the fingers will be able to straighten and move more freely, which will improve hand function. The majority of patients state that their quality of life has been greatly improved by their increased capacity to carry out routine actions like typing, shaking hands, and holding objects.

Successful surgery can result in a long-lasting improvement in the appearance and functionality of the hands. While the rate of contracture recurrence varies, surgical therapies typically have a lower rate of recurrence than less invasive treatments. The long-term effects on hand function and mobility highlight the possible advantages of choosing surgical treatment.

Alternative Medical Therapies And Their Performance

For the management of Dupuytren's Contracture, there are several non-surgical options available, each with differing degrees of effectiveness. Collagenase clostridium histolyticum (Xiaflex) injections and needle aponeurotomy (needle fasciotomy) are examples of non-surgical alternatives. By puncturing and breaking the tissue cords causing the contracture with a needle, a procedure known as needle aponeurotomy can offer instant, but frequently transient, relief.

By enzymatically dissolving the constricted tissue, collagenase injections enable the finger to straighten. For more severe or advanced cases of Dupuytren's Contracture, these less invasive and quicker-to-recover techniques might not work as well. Furthermore, compared to surgery, these treatments may have greater rates of recurrence. Patients are better able to make decisions regarding their care when they are aware of the benefits and drawbacks of each option.

Testimonials And Patient Satisfaction Rates

Dupuytren's Contracture surgery typically has high patient satisfaction ratings, which attests to the procedure's efficacy in regaining hand function and minimizing discomfort.

Following surgery, many patients express relief and thankfulness for their increased mobility and decreased discomfort. Testimonials frequently emphasize the beneficial effects on day-to-day activities and general quality of life.

For example, many patients report being able to resume activities and jobs that the contract had previously made difficult. Success examples highlight the importance of well-trained surgical teams and thorough care plans in producing positive results. These first-hand experiences show that there is hope for a successful surgical outcome and offer comfort and understanding to others who are thinking about the treatment.

The Value Of Continued Care

An essential element of a successful Dupuytren's Contracture surgical procedure is follow-up treatment. Hand exercises and physical therapy are important components of post-operative rehabilitation that help to maximize the advantages of surgery and minimize problems.

Scheduling routine follow-up meetings with the surgeon enables early identification of any problems and monitoring of the healing process.

Patients are frequently instructed on particular exercises to keep their fingers strong and flexible. Following these recommendations can greatly improve healing and reduce the chance of contracture recurrence.

Education on wound care, infection symptoms, and appropriate hand ergonomics contributes to a more seamless recuperation process. Making sure patients receive thorough follow-up care enables them to benefit as much as possible from their operation.

CHAPTER FIVE

RESTORATION AS WELL AS RECOVERY

Quick Postoperative Treatment

Patients undergoing surgery for Dupuytren's contracture usually spend a little time in the recovery room after the procedure so that medical personnel may keep an eye on their vital signs and make sure there are no aftereffects from the anesthesia or surgery. The hand may be raised to lessen swelling during this period, and the surgical site will be covered with a sterile bandage.

To reduce swelling and encourage healing, it is essential to keep the hand as elevated as possible for the first 24 to 48 hours following surgery. You can also apply ice packs on and off to manage discomfort and swelling.

Patients will typically receive detailed instructions on how to take care of the surgical site, which will include cleaning and drying the bandage. It's critical to keep the bandage dry to avoid infection. Should stitches be utilized, they might require drying out until they are taken out, which often happens 10–14 days after surgery. To keep the fingers straight and stop them from constricting during the first healing phase, a splint may be used in some situations.

Exercises And Physical Therapy

A vital part of the recovery process after Dupuytren's contracture surgery is physical therapy. A physical therapist will usually create an exercise plan specifically designed to help the hand and fingers regain strength and movement. Typically, these activities start mildly and get more intense as the healing process goes on. To increase strength and flexibility, common workouts include bending, gripping, and finger stretching.

To get the best results possible, physical therapy must be participated in on a regular and consistent basis. Apart from their regular therapy sessions, patients could be directed to undertake specific exercises multiple times a day at their residences. This encourages the restoration of normal function and aids in the prevention of scar tissue from developing. It's critical to carefully follow the therapist's directions and avoid overdoing the workouts, as this may result in difficulties or setbacks.

Techniques For Pain Management

An essential part of healing following Dupuytren's contracture surgery is pain control. To alleviate pain in the days after surgery, doctors frequently prescribe patients acetaminophen or nonsteroidal anti-inflammatory medicines (NSAIDs). Stronger painkillers might be required in some situations for a brief amount of time. It's critical to take these drugs as directed by your doctor and to let them know if your pain is not being managed.

Apart from pharmaceuticals, alternative approaches to managing pain may also prove beneficial. These could include employing elevation to lessen swelling, applying ice to the injured area, and engaging in relaxation exercises like deep breathing or meditation. By increasing blood flow and lowering hand and finger rigidity, physical therapy can help control pain as well.

Going Back To Work And Daily Activities

Depending on the patient and the complexity of the procedure, there may be a different time frame for going back to regular activities and employment. After surgery, most patients can usually resume modest activities a few days to a week later, though they may need to avoid occupations requiring a strong grip or heavy hand usage for many weeks.

whether it comes to knowing whether it is safe to go back to work, patients should heed their surgeon's recommendations, particularly if their line of employment requires manual labor or repeated hand movements. During the initial phase of rehabilitation, work obligations may need to be modified in certain instances. It's crucial to stay away from activities that can put stress on the hand and impede the healing process.

Tracking Development And Possible Issues

Maintaining regular follow-up meetings with the surgeon is crucial for tracking the healing process and addressing any issues that may arise.

The surgeon will look for indications of complications including infection, excessive edema, or problems healing the wound during these visits.

At home, patients should be on the lookout for any indications of complications, such as increased redness, swelling, discomfort, or discharge from the surgery site, and they should promptly report any such signals to their healthcare physician.

In certain instances, if the contracture starts to reoccur or if there are problems with the initial surgical result, other therapies like steroid injections or additional surgery can be required.

Maintaining regular contact with your medical team and following rehabilitation guidelines are essential to a full recovery and lowering the possibility of problems.

CHAPTER SIX

CHANGES IN LIFESTYLE POSSIBLE FOR DUPUYTREN'S CONTRACTION

Keeping Dupuytren's Contracture From Recurring

A proactive strategy is needed to stop Dupuytren's contract from recurring. Regularly extending your hands and fingers is an important tactic.

These exercises assist in preserving flexibility and guard against the accumulation of scar tissue, which can result in contractures.

Additionally, it's critical to keep an eye out for any recurrence of the problem, including lumps or tightness in the palm. If these symptoms manifest, get medical attention.

You can lessen the strain on your hands by avoiding heavy gripping chores and repetitive hand motions. If these kinds of tasks are part of your job or your interests, think about taking regular pauses to stretch and decompress your hands. Reducing hand strain can also be achieved by wearing supporting gloves and adopting good hand ergonomics.

Hand Use Ergonomic Considerations

To manage Dupuytren's contracture and stop its progression, ergonomics is essential. Make sure your workspace is configured to facilitate natural hand positions, which will lessen needless strain.

For example, when using a computer, utilize a strain-reduction keyboard and mouse and maintain a neutral wrist position.

Tools and equipment used in the workplace should be chosen and modified so that your hands can comfortably fit them. Handles and grips with ergonomic designs can greatly lessen the strain on the fingers and palm.

Furthermore, minimizing strain and preventing the worsening of symptoms can be achieved by learning and putting into practice appropriate lifting techniques and hand postures.

Tools And Adaptive Aids For Daily Tasks

You can make chores easier and more pleasant by including adaptive tools and aids in your daily routine. Many gadgets, like ergonomic culinary utensils, button hooks, and jar openers, are made to help with hand function.

The purpose of these gadgets is to lessen the need for very tight grasping and twisting movements, which can make Dupuytren's contracture worse.

To minimize the necessity for recurrent hand movements, take into consideration utilizing voice-activated devices and touch-free technology.

With the help of adaptive aids, you may carry out daily duties more comfortably and independently, which can significantly enhance your quality of life.

Including Hand Exercises In Everyday Activities

For the hands to remain flexible and functional, regular hand workouts are essential. You can do basic stretches several times a day, including gently bending and straightening your fingers.

These workouts lower the chance of contractures and maintain the suppleness of the hand's tissues.

It's simple to incorporate these exercises into your everyday regimen. You can complete them, for instance, before bed, during work breaks, or while watching TV. Maintaining consistency is essential; even a little daily stretch session can have a big impact over time.

Lifestyle And Dietary Factors Affecting Hand Health

In addition to supporting hand health, leading a healthy lifestyle can potentially halt the advancement of Dupuytren's contracture.

Fruits, vegetables, nuts, seafood, and other foods high in anti-inflammatory components can help lower inflammation and improve tissue health in general.

It's crucial to stay hydrated, abstain from excessive alcohol use, and quit smoking because these behaviors can have a detrimental impact on tissue health and blood flow. Your hands will feel less strain if you maintain a healthy weight and engage in regular physical activity.

By implementing these lifestyle changes, you can improve hand health and manage Dupuytren's contracture more easily, all while preserving your standard of living.

CHAPTER SEVEN

THE PSYCHOLOGICAL AND EMOTIONAL ASPECTS OF DUPUYTREN'S FRACTURE SURGERY

Handling Stress And Anxiety Before Surgery

It's normal to feel worried in the days before surgery because it can be a frightening experience. Learning everything you can about the operation and its advantages will help you better handle these emotions.

Fear can be minimized and the procedure demystified by knowing what to anticipate. Mindfulness meditation, deep breathing techniques, and mild physical activities like yoga or walking can all aid in mental relaxation.

Speaking with a trusted friend, relative, or counselor about their fears can be beneficial for certain patients.

Furthermore, a sense of control and stress reduction can be achieved by making sure that all logistical parts of the surgery day are adequately organized.

Effects On Confidence And Self-Image

Self-image and confidence can be severely impacted by Dupuytren's contracture, a disorder that affects the appearance and function of the hand. Some people might feel self-conscious about the alterations in their hands' look.

There may be temporary swelling or visible scars after surgery, which can potentially alter your self-perception.

It's critical to keep in mind that these modifications are a normal aspect of the healing process and get better with time.

Keeping an optimistic attitude and concentrating on the functional gains made possible by the operation might help lessen unpleasant emotions.

Confidence-boosting activities like hobbies and social events can also be quite important for regaining self-esteem.

Systems And Resources For Assistance Offered

Systems of support are essential both before and after surgery. The healing process goes more smoothly when friends, family, and support groups are there to offer both practical and emotional support.

Getting involved in a support group for people with Dupuytren's contracture can provide a feeling of camaraderie and common ground.

Local groups and internet forums can provide resources and guidance from people who have experienced comparable procedures.

If patients want further emotional assistance, mental health specialists might be contacted by healthcare practitioners.

By making use of these tools, you can share your struggles and victories with like-minded people and avoid feeling alone on your journey.

Taking Care Of Fears And Concerns

It's normal to be afraid about surgery and to worry about things like pain, recuperation time, or the result.

Talking openly with your surgical team is the best approach to address these anxieties.

Inquire about the process, anesthetic, pain relief, and what to anticipate from the healing period. Comprehending the procedural aspects and the probability of distinct results might offer comfort.

Speaking with a mental health expert about any particular anxiety is also beneficial, as they can offer coping mechanisms that are customized to your needs.

You can change your perspective from one of worry to one of optimism by envisioning a successful result and emphasizing the positive features of the surgery.

A Look At Mental Health Issues During Rehabilitation

Following surgery, recovery is a dual process that involves both physical and mental aspects. It's critical to practice self-compassion and acknowledge that experiencing emotional highs and lows is common. Remaining socially connected and participating in light activities can help prevent feelings of loneliness.

Do not be reluctant to seek professional mental health assistance if you experience anxiety or depression during your recovery.

Maintaining a journal of your healing process can also give you a constructive way to express your ideas and emotions, which will enable you to monitor your progress and establish reasonable objectives for your recovery. Remind yourself that maintaining your mental well-being is just as important as your physical recovery.

CHAPTER EIGHT

PATIENT EXPERIENCES AND CASE STUDIES

True Accounts Of People With Dupuytren's

Numerous individuals worldwide are impacted by Dupuytren's contracture, and each has a distinct tale to tell. John, a 55-year-old carpenter, for example, began to notice a progressive tightening in his right hand.

His fingers eventually bent toward his palm, making it difficult for him to grip the equipment. John was first indifferent to the condition and only went to the doctor when it was seriously interfering with his career.

In a similar vein, Mary, a 60-year-old retired teacher, discovered that her love of gardening was being thwarted by her fingers' increasing constriction.

Although both people had surgery, their experiences and results were different.

Different Surgical Journeys And Outcomes

John had a successful surgery. His hand was fully functional again after the fasciectomy treatment, which involved removing the swollen tissue. With the help of physical therapy, he recovered quickly and was back to work in a few months.

Mary's voyage, on the other hand, was more intricate. She had the same treatment, but because she was older and her body healed more slowly, she had problems.

Her recuperation was longer than expected, necessitating more treatments like occupational therapy and regular check-ups. These disparate results emphasize the variation in Dupuytren's contracture patients' surgical success and recuperation periods.

Lessons Discovered From Various Situations

John and Mary's experiences highlight several important lessons. First, better results may result from early intervention. John's prompt choice to seek medical attention made for a simple surgical procedure and a speedy recovery. However, Mary's inaction led to a more difficult and drawn-out recuperation process. The importance of postoperative care is yet another crucial lesson. Physical and occupational therapy was very beneficial to both patients and was very important to their recovery. These instances also demonstrate the important role that age and general health play in determining surgical outcomes.

Perspectives From Medical Experts

When treating Dupuytren's contracture, medical experts stress the value of a multidisciplinary approach. To guarantee the greatest results for patients, surgeons collaborate with physical therapists and occupational therapists.

Hand surgeon Dr. Smith emphasizes the need to have reasonable expectations. Professional advice from physical therapist Jane Doe emphasizes the teamwork needed to effectively manage Dupuytren's contracture. "Patients need to understand that while surgery can significantly improve function, it may not completely restore it to pre-condition levels." "Consistent and targeted exercises post-surgery are essential for regaining mobility and strength."

Useful Suggestions Based On Patient Input

Several useful suggestions are revealed, based on comments from patients who have had surgery to treat Dupuytren's contracture. Initially, individuals advise consulting a doctor as soon as symptoms start to manifest.

Severe contractures can be avoided and easier surgical operations can result from early diagnosis and treatment.

Secondly, it is imperative to comply with postoperative care protocols, which include the recommended exercises. Patients such as John and Mary discovered that regular follow-up with physical therapy had a major impact on their healing. Finally, keeping lines of communication open with medical professionals on discomfort, development, and any worries can assist in quickly addressing problems and modifying treatment plans as necessary.

CHAPTER NINE

FAQS AND REGULAR QUESTIONS

What Leads To The Contracture Of Dupuytren?

The disorder known as Dupuytren's contracture mainly affects the hands, causing the fibrous tissue that lies beneath the skin of the fingers and palm to thicken and shrink. Although the precise etiology of Dupuytren's contracture is still unknown, a mix of environmental and genetic variables is thought to play a role. Significantly raising the risk in the event of a family history of the illness implies a hereditary component. It also happens more often in men than in women and is more prevalent in people of Northern European ancestry. Dupuytren's contracture has also been connected to environmental variables including drinking alcohol and smoking, as well as certain medical disorders like diabetes. The illness usually develops gradually over several years, starting with little nodules or lumps in the palm and progressing to more severe contractures that restrict the movement of the fingers.

How Can I Tell Whether I Need Surgery?

Dupuytren's contracture severity and impact on everyday activities must be considered when deciding whether surgery is required. Gentle situations that don't affect hand function could be treated with observation or non-surgical therapies rather than surgery. Surgery might be necessary, though, if the contracture gets to the point where it makes it difficult to carry out daily activities including shaking hands, buttoning clothes, or holding objects. The right course of action will be determined by a complete evaluation by a healthcare professional, which frequently includes tests to quantify the degree of contracture and hand function. When conservative measures have failed and the contracture significantly reduces hand function and quality of life, surgery is usually recommended.

Dupuytren's contracture can be managed non-surgically in several ways, especially in the early stages. Among these substitutes are:

Needle aponeurotomy (NA): This minimally invasive technique entails puncturing and breaking the thicker tissue cords with a needle to release the contracture. Compared to standard surgery, it has less recovery time and is carried out under local anesthesia.

Collagenase Injections: To break down the collagen buildup, an enzyme known as collagenase can be injected into the afflicted tissue. Manual hand manipulation is typically used to extend and straighten the fingers after this treatment.

Physical treatment: While less successful in treating advanced contractures, hand therapy exercises can assist preserve function and mobility.

Splitting:

Especially at night, wearing a splint can assist in maintaining finger extension and delay the contracture's advancement.

Every one of these options has advantages and disadvantages of its own. Based on the patient's general health and the severity of the ailment, a healthcare professional can assist in determining the best course of action.

How Much Time Does Recovery Take After Surgery?

The length of recovery following surgery for Dupuytren's contracture varies based on the degree of the procedure and the patient's general condition. Patients should typically anticipate a few weeks to several months for complete recovery. The hand will be bandaged immediately after surgery, and a splint may be required to keep the fingers straight. In the early postoperative days following surgery, discomfort and edema are usual, and the medical team will offer pain management techniques.

Rehabilitation through physical therapy is essential for regaining hand strength and flexibility. Gentle hand exercises are often recommended for patients to begin as soon as surgery to promote recovery and avoid stiffness. Scheduling routine follow-up visits with the surgeon will guarantee that the healing process is proceeding as planned and that any difficulties are dealt with as soon as possible. Following the recommended rehabilitation program is crucial to getting the best results.

What Kind Of Hand Function Can I Expect Following Surgery?

Following surgery, hand function improves significantly for the majority of patients, with many being able to perform formerly difficult daily tasks again. The degree of functional recovery may differ depending on the type of surgery done and how severe the contracture was before surgery.

As the hand recovers, patients may initially have some stiffness or limited movement; however, these symptoms usually get better with time and physical therapy. To optimize healing, it's critical to adhere to the therapist's and surgeon's instructions for post-operative care and exercise. Minor residual stiffness or decreased range of motion may occasionally endure, but these are often negligible in comparison to the state before surgery.

Improving the quality of life and restoring as much normal function as feasible are the long-term objectives of surgery. Dupuytren's contracture can reoccur, however many patients experience years of better hand function before requiring additional therapy. Maintaining ideal hand health can be facilitated by aggressive therapy of any early indications of recurrence and routine monitoring.